# The Definitive Vegetaria

CW00508114

## A Set of Super Affordable and Easy to Make Recipes for Any Occasion to Lose Weight

Skye Webb

# Table of contents

# Artichoke and Spinach Salad

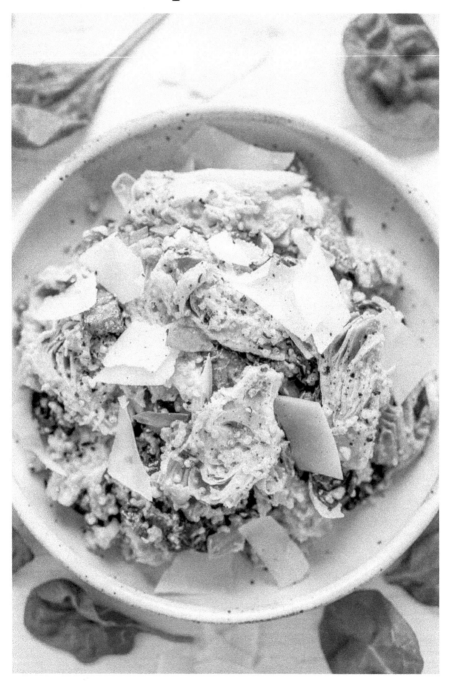

Preparation time: 5 minutes Cooking time: 0 minutes Servings: 4

Ingredients:

2        tablespoons avocado oil

2 garlic cloves, minced

2 tablespoons cilantro, chopped

14 ounces canned artichokes, drained and halved

2 cups baby spinach, chopped

½ cup cucumber, roughly cubed

½ teaspoon basil, dried

Salt and black pepper to the taste

Directions:

1. In a bowl, combine the artichokes with the garlic, the oil and the other ingredients, toss, divide into smaller bowls and serve as an appetizer.

Nutrition: calories 223, fat 11.2, fiber 5.34, carbs 15.5, protein 7.4

# Red Pepper and Cheese Dip

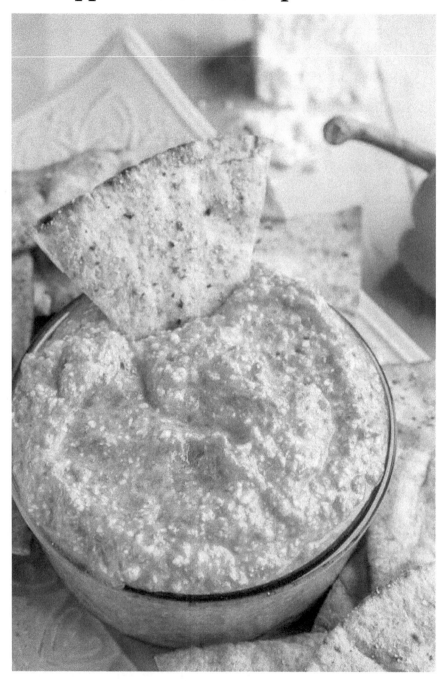

Preparation time: 10 minutes Cooking time: 10 minutes

Servings: 4

Ingredients:

7 ounces roasted red peppers, chopped

½ cup cashew cheese, grated

2 tablespoons parsley, chopped

2 tablespoons olive oil

¼ cup capers, drained

1 tablespoon lemon juice

Directions:

1.     Heat up a pan with the oil over medium heat, add the peppers and the other ingredients, stir, cook for 10 minutes and take off the heat.

2.     Blend using an immersion blender, divide the mix into bowls and serve.

Nutrition: calories 95, fat 8.6, fiber 1.2, carbs 4.7, protein 1.4

# Mushroom Falafel

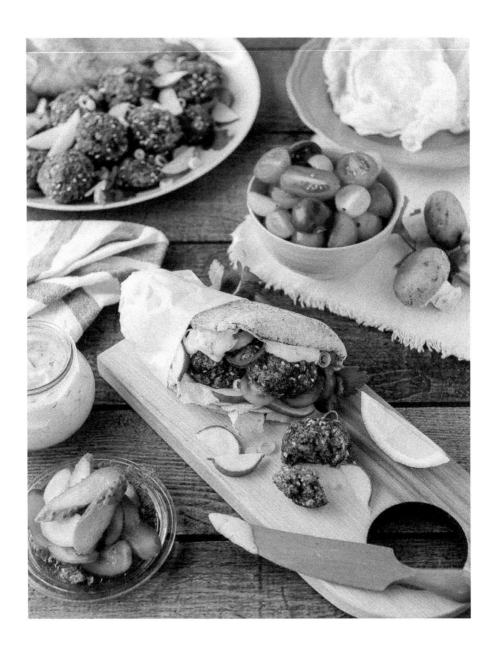

Preparation time: 10 minutes Cooking time: 12 minutes Servings: 6

Ingredients:

1 cup mushrooms, chopped

1 bunch parsley leaves

4    scallions, hopped

5    garlic cloves, minced

1 teaspoon coriander, ground

A pinch of salt and black pepper

¼ teaspoon baking soda

1 teaspoon lemon juice

3 tablespoons almond flour

2 tablespoons avocado oil

Directions:

1.    In your food processor, combine the mushrooms with the parsley and the other ingredients except the flour and the oil and pulse well.

2.    Transfer the mix to a bowl, add the flour, stir well, shape medium balls out of this mix and flatten them a bit.

3.    Heat up a pan with the over medium-high heat, add the falafels, cook them for 6 minutes on each side, drain excess grease using paper towels, arrange them on a platter and serve as an appetizer.

Nutrition: calories 55, fat 3.5, fiber 1.5, carbs 4.5, protein 2.3

# Baked Hot Spicy Cashews Snack

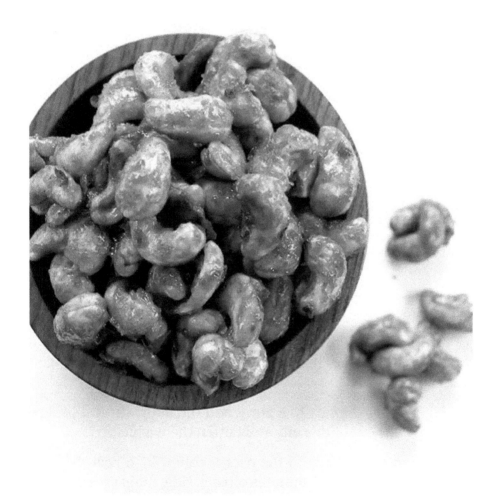

Preparation Time: 20 minutes Cooking Time: 35 minutes Servings: 8

Ingredients:

2½ c. raw cashews

1/3 c. olive oil

½ tsp. turmeric powder

1 tsp. garlic powder

3 c. hot pepper sauce

Directions:

1.      In a mixing bowl, mix hot pepper sauce, oil and stir in the turmeric and garlic powder.

2.      Add the cashews to the bowl and completely coat with hot pepper sauce mixture.

3.      Soak cashews in the hot sauce mixture for several hours.

4.      Preheat oven to 325F.

5.      Spread the cashews onto a baking sheet and bake for 35-35 minutes.

6.      Allow cool and serve.

Nutrition: Calories: 41, Fat: 29.01g, Carbs: 9.6g, Protein: 6.71g

# Easy Avocado and Cremini Mushroom Melts

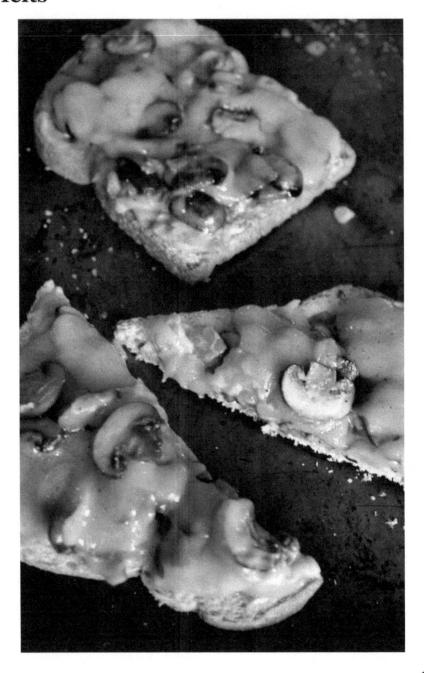

Preparation Time: 15 minutes Cooking Time: 25 minutes Servings: 4

Ingredients:

8 sliced Cremini mushrooms

1 tbsp. olive oil

1 c. guacamole

1 tbsp. balsamic vinegar

12 slices cheddar cheese

3 slices Keto bread

Salt Pepper

Directions:

1.      Preheat oven to 350°F.

2.      Using a skillet, Sauté balsamic vinegar, mushrooms, and olive oil medium high heat for 15 minutes, as you stir oftenly, until mushrooms are fragrant and golden brown.

3.      Spread guacamole on bread and top with sautéed cheese and mushrooms.

4.      Bake for approximately 10 minutes and ensure all the cheese melts out.

5.      Serve and enjoy!

Nutrition: Calories: 77, Fat: 16.25g, Carbs: 11.35g, Protein: 9.32g

# Keto Hot Peppers C.s

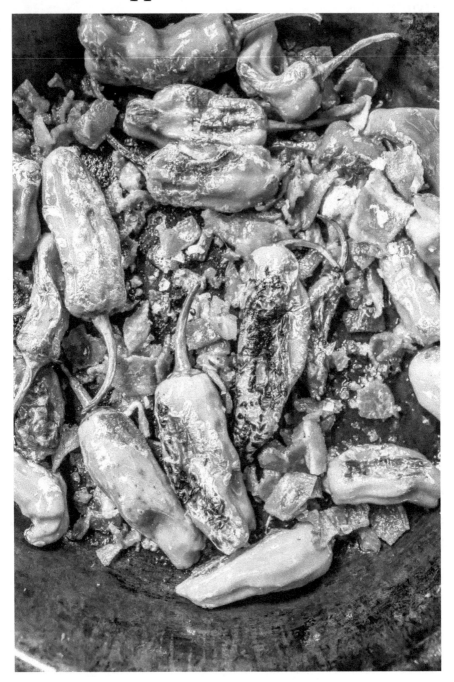

Preparation Time: 15 minutes Cooking Time: 15-20 minutes Servings: 4

Ingredients

4 eggs, beaten

3       hot red peppers, dried

8 tbsps. buckwheat flour

2 tsps. baking powder

2½ tbsps. coconut milk

4       freshly chopped basil leaves

1 tbsp. olive oil

½ tsp. salt

Directions:

1.      Preheat oven to 380F.

2.      In a bowl, mix the eggs, coconut milk, fresh basil and hot peppers.

3.      In a separate mixing bowl, mix the buckwheat flour with the baking powder and salt.

4.      Unite the egg mixture with the flour mixture and stir well.

5.      Pour the batter in cups (3/4 c. full).

6.      Bake in oven for 15-20 minutes.

7.      When ready let cool and serve.

Nutrition: Calories: 35, Fat: 11.65g, Carbs: 16.33g, Protein: 12.57g

# Spanish Vegetable Omelet

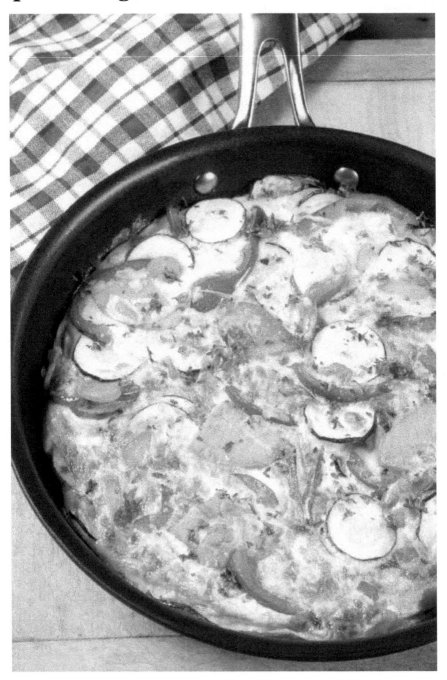

Preparation Time: 10 minutes Cooking Time: 15 minutes

Servings: 4


Ingredients:

6 eggs

2 red peppers, chopped in thin strips

3 tbsps. olive oil

2 chopped scallions

1 diced zucchini

Salt

Black pepper


Directions:

1.      Heat the olive oil in a pan; sauté chopped green onions for 3-4 minutes.

2.      Add the peppers and cook for about 2 minutes more.

3.      Add the zucchini and sauté for another 3 minutes.

4.      In a mixing bowl, beat the eggs. Add salt and pepper to taste.

5.      Mix the vegetables into the eggs.

6.      Heat the olive oil in the frying pan and pour the whisked eggs mixture into the skillet.

7.      Cook the omelet for 1 to 2 minutes. Serve hot.

Nutrition: Calories: 0, Fat: 7.53g, Carbs: 6.7, Protein: 10.91g

# Absolute Avocado Pizza

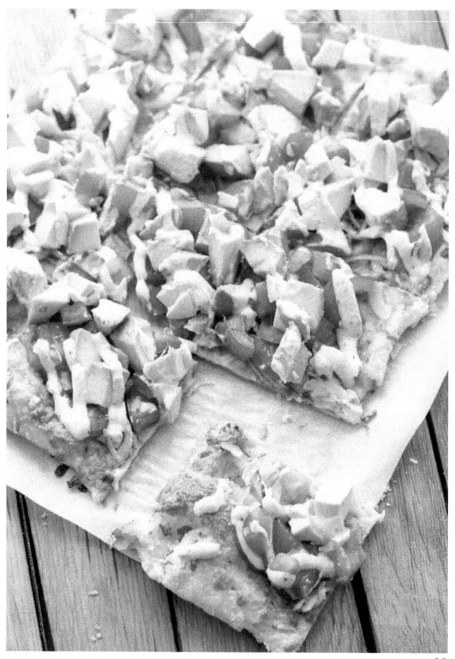

Preparation Time: 10 minutes Cooking Time: 25 minutes Servings: 4

Ingredients:

Dough 2 eggs

4 tbsps. grated Parmesan cheese

2 envelopes unflavored gelatin

½ c. unsweetened

Greek yogurt

4 tbsps. water

3 tbsps. grass-fed butter

Salt

Filling

Cheese, mushrooms, avocado puree, chopped fresh parsley

Directions:

1.    Preheat oven to 450 degrees F.

2.    Place all ingredients in a blender (gelatin without dissolving and beat well.

3.    Grease a parchment paper with butter and evenly distribute the dough.

4.    Place dough in greased baking pan and bake about 15 minutes.

5.    Remove pizza from the oven and spread evenly with avocado sauce.

6. Top with your favorite fillings and sprinkle with the cheese.

7. Bake for 5 -10 minutes.

8. Remove from oven, let rest for 5 minutes and slice.

9. Serve immediately.

Nutrition: Calories: 65, Fat: 20.87g, Carbs: 1.22g, Protein: 18.27g

# Almond Lemon Biscuits

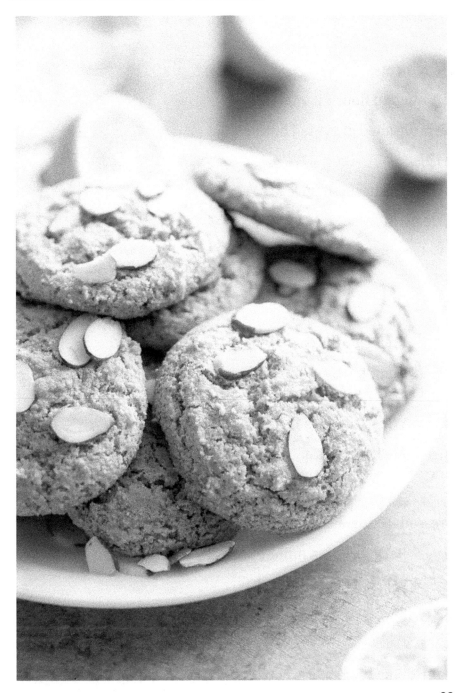

Preparation Time: 10 minutes Cooking Time: 12-15 minutes Servings: 6

Ingredients:

3 c. almond flour

½ c. unsalted grass-fed butter

2 eggs

1 tbsp. fresh lemon juice

3 tbsps. Stevia

1½ tsps. Baking powder

Directions:

1.    Preheat oven to 350F.

2.    Combine the almond flour, Stevia and baking powder in a bowl.

3.    Whisk the eggs in a separate bowl.

4.    Melt the butter, and combine with almond flour, lemon juice and eggs mixture; stir well.

5.    Divide mixture equally into 6 biscuits and place in a greased baking dish.

6.    Bake for 12-15 minutes.

7.    Let cool on a wire rack.

8.    Serve warm or cold.

Nutrition: Calories: 27, Fat: 25.91g, Carbs: 4.49g, Protein 5.9g

# Cherry shed Coconut Muffins

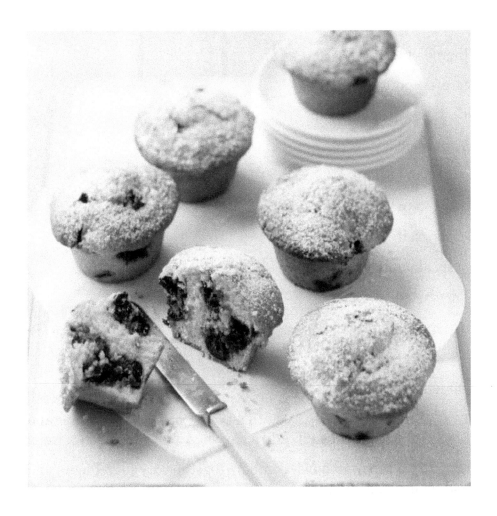

Preparation Time: 15 minutes Cooking Time: 30 minutes Servings: 12

Ingredients:

½ c. coconut oil

1       c. coconut sugar

½ mashed avocado

2 c. coconut flour

2       tsps. Baking powder

½ tsp. salt

1 tsp. almond extract

1 c. toasted almonds

2 c. chopped cherries

Directions:

1.      Preheat oven to 375°F. In a bowl, beat coconut butter and Stevia (or coconut sugar). Add a smashed avocado and mix well.

2.      In a separate bowl, combine together dry ingredients and add them to the mixture.

3.      Stir in almond extract, almonds and cherries.

4.      Pour muffin batter into 12 greased muffin cups.

5.      Bake muffins for 30 minutes.

6.      Serve warm or cold.

Nutrition: Calories: 7, Fat: 14.82g, Carbs: 5.79g, Protein: 2.89g

# Creamy Blackberry Cinnamon Smoothie

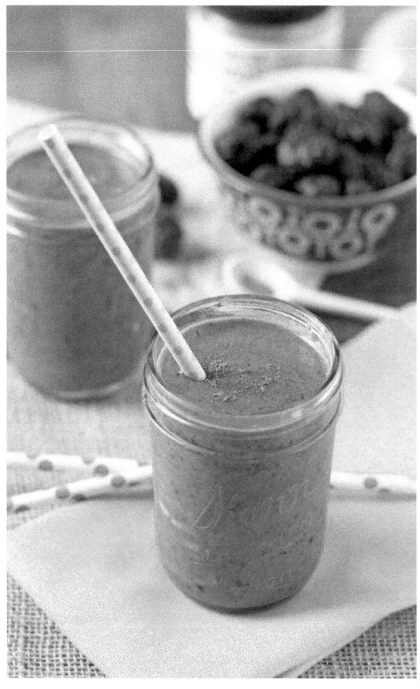

Preparation Time: 3 minutes Cooking Time: 0 minutes Servings: 3

Ingredients

1 c. frozen blackberries

1 c. unsweetened vanilla almond milk

½ c. full fat vanilla yogurt

2 tsp. ground cinnamon

1 tbsp. arrowroot powder

1 tsp. pure vanilla extract

½ c. water

Directions:

1.      Place all ingredients from the list in your high-speed blender.

2.      Blend until smooth and creamy.

3.      Decorate with fresh or frozen blackberries and serve.

4.      Enjoy!

Nutrition: Calories: 83.78, Fat: 1.42g, Carbs: 8.56g, Protein: 2.97g

# Dark Coco-Almond Bars

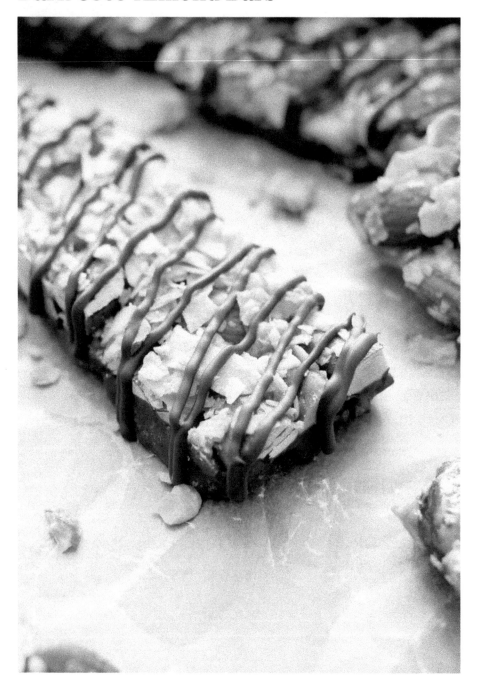

Preparation Time: 10 minutes Cooking Time: 0 minutes

Servings: 12

Ingredients:

1       c. shredded coconut

1 c. almond butter

2       c. raw almonds (preferably peeled ones)

1 tbsp. coconut flour

1 c. melted coconut oil

1½ tbsp. Stevia

3 oz. dark chocolate

1       tbsp. organic vanilla extract Salt

Directions:

1.      Place almonds in your blender, close the lid, and blend on High for 10 seconds.

2.      Pour all of the remaining ingredients, except the chocolate, and pulse until it forms a textured paste.

3.      Line a baking sheet with parchment paper.

4.      Pour the mixture into pan and lightly press to smooth out.

5.      Refrigerate for about 2 hours, until set.

6.      Melt the chocolate over a bain-marie (double boiler), and spread it over the bars, smoothing out with spatula until evenly coated.

7.	Place back into the refrigerator for about 30 minutes, until the chocolate is set.

8.	Cut into 12 bars and serve!


Nutrition: Calories: 46, Fat: 30.62g, Carbs: 7.69g, Protein: 7.5g

# Keto Almond Zucchini Bread

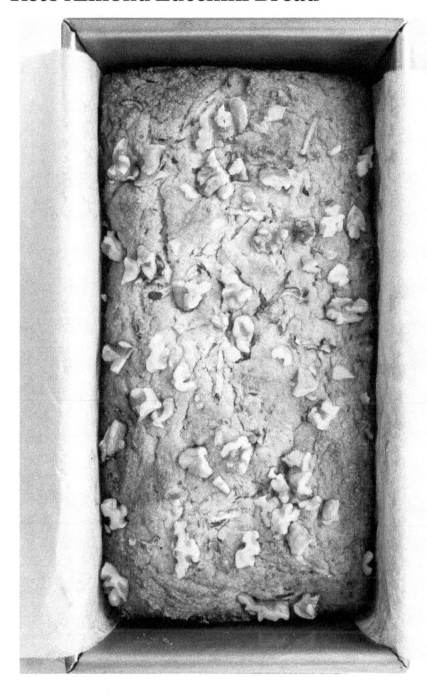

Preparation Time: 15 minutes Cooking Time: 35 minutes Servings: 8

Ingredients:

2      eggs

1 c. zucchini, grated

1½ c. almond flour

1 c. chopped almonds

¾ c. Stevia

1 tbsp. ground cinnamon

1 tsp. pure vanilla extract

2 tbsps. coconut oil

1 tsp. baking soda

Salt

Directions:

1.      Preheat oven to 360F degrees.

2.      Grease a loaf pan with melted coconut oil and set aside.

3.      Whisk the eggs, organic vanilla extract, coconut oil and Stevia in a bowl.

4.      With the help of an electric mixer, beat the egg mixture until combined well.

5.      Add the almond flour, baking soda, salt and ground cinnamon and continue to mix.

6.      Add in grated zucchini and chopped almonds and mix again until all ingredients combined well.

7.      Pour the mixture in a prepared loaf pan and bake for 35 minutes.

8.      Let cool for 10 minutes, slice and serve.


Nutrition: Calories: 33, Fat: 7.27g, Carbs: 8.58g, Protein: 4.78g

# Light Cabbage Mayo Salad

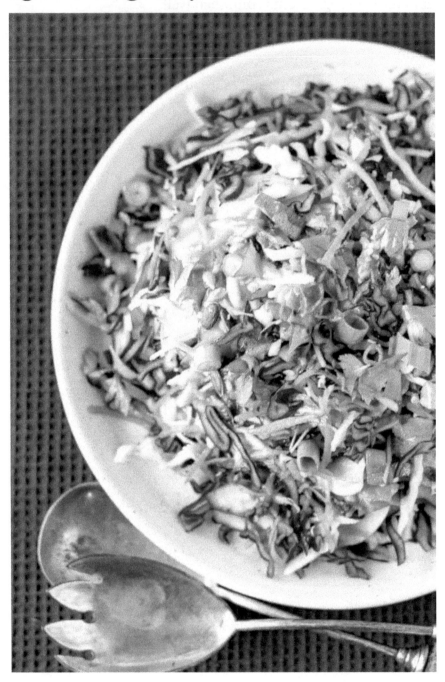

Preparation Time: 5 minutes Cooking Time: 0 minutes Servings: 2

Ingredients

½ medium cabbage head

Salt

¼ c. Mayonnaise gluten-free, grain free

2 tbsps. Cheddar cheese

Directions:

1.      Wash your cabbage and rinse. The outermost leaves should be removed.

2.      Half the cabbage and chop.

3.      Place the cabbage in large container and season with salt.

4.      Pour mayonnaise and stir well.

5.      You can refrigerate salad about one hour before serving.

6.      Sprinkle with Cheddar cheese if used and serve.

Nutrition: Calories: 99.59, Fat: 3.62g, Carbs: 6.86g, Protein: 5.33g

# Peppermint-Cilantro Artichoke Hearts

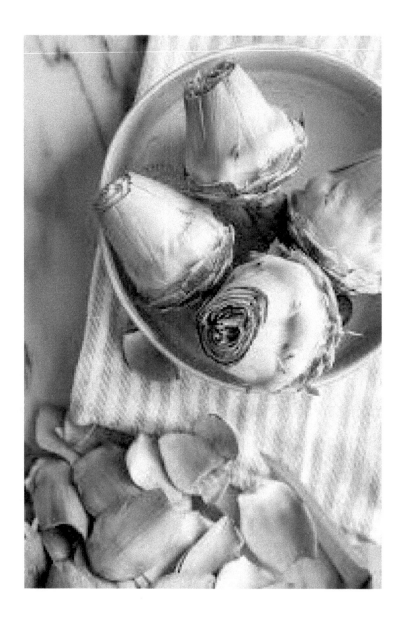

Preparation Time: 10 minutes Cooking Time: 20 minutes Servings: 4

Ingredients:

6 artichoke hearts

4 minced garlic cloves

3 c. water

4 tbsps. Extra-virgin olive oil

3 tbsps. Chopped peppermint leaves 3

 tbsps. Chopped cilantro leaves

2 tbsps. Lemon juice

Salt

Black pepper

Directions:

1.     In a deep pan place cleaned artichokes along with water, oil, cilantro leaves, peppermint, lemon juice, and garlic.

2.     Season salt and pepper to taste and bring to a boil.

3.     Reduce heat and simmer artichokes about 15–20 minutes, turning occasionally.

4.     Transfer artichokes to a serving platter and drizzle with some of the cooking liquid.

5.     Serve.

Nutrition: Calories: 33, Fat: 13.77g, Carbs: 9.47g, Protein: 5.48

# Brussels sprouts Chips

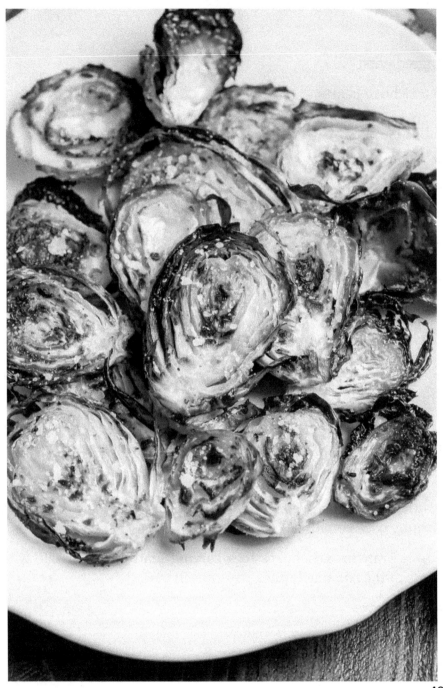

Preparation Time: 10 minutes Cooking Time: 10 minutes Servings: 2

Ingredients

10 Brussels sprouts split leaves

1 tbsp. olive oil

¼ tsp. sea salt

Directions:

1.      Preheat your oven to 350˚ Fahrenheit.

2.      Toss Brussels sprouts with olive oil.

3.      Season Brussels sprouts with salt. Spread Brussels sprouts in a baking dish and bake in preheated oven for 10 minutes.

4.      Serve and enjoy!

Nutrition: Calories: 101, Fat: 7.3g, Cabs: 8.6g, Protein: 3.2g

# Zaatar Popcorn

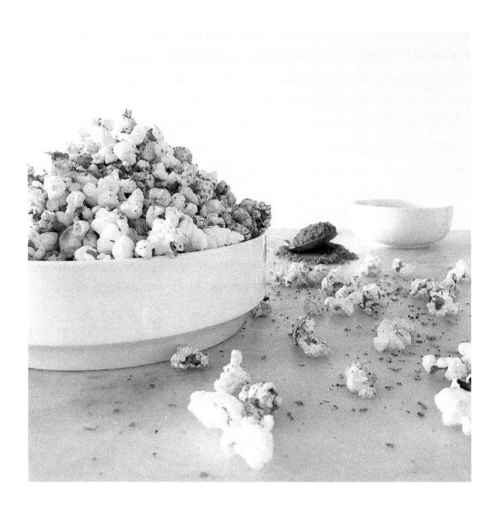

Preparation Time: 10 minutes Cooking Time: 0 minute Servings: 8

Ingredients:

8 cups popped popcorns

1/4 cup za'atar spice blend

¾ teaspoon salt

4 tablespoons olive oil

Directions:

1.      Place all the ingredients except for popcorns in a large bowl and whisk until combined.

2.      Then add popcorns, toss until well coated, and serve straight away.

Nutrition: Calories:150 Cal, Fat: 9 g, Carbs: 15 g, Protein: 2 g, Fiber: 4 g

# Potato Chips

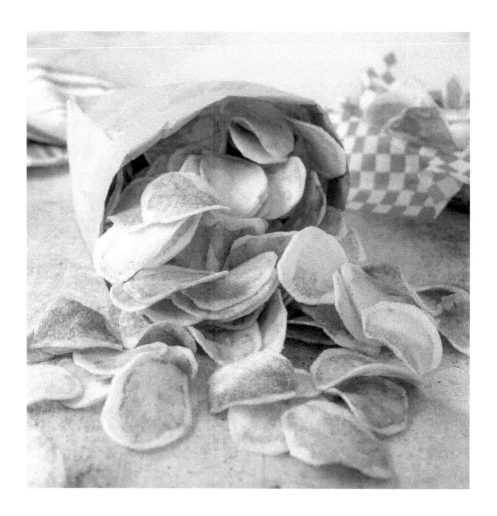

Preparation Time: 10 minutes Cooking Time: 20 minutes Servings: 2

Ingredients:

3 medium potatoes, scrubbed, thinly sliced, soaked in warm water for 10 min

½ teaspoon garlic powder

½ teaspoon onion powder

½ teaspoon red chili powder

½ teaspoon curry powder

1 teaspoon of sea salt

1 tablespoon apple cider vinegar

2 tablespoons olive oil

Direction:

1.     Drain the potato slices, pat dry, then place them in a large bowl, add remaining ingredients and toss until well coated.

2.     Spread the potatoes in a single layer on a baking sheet and bake for 20 minutes until crispy, turning halfway.

3.     Serve straight away.

Nutrition: Calories: 600 Cal, Fat: 30 g, Carbs: 78 g, Protein: 9 g, Fiber: 23 g

# Spinach and Artichoke Dip

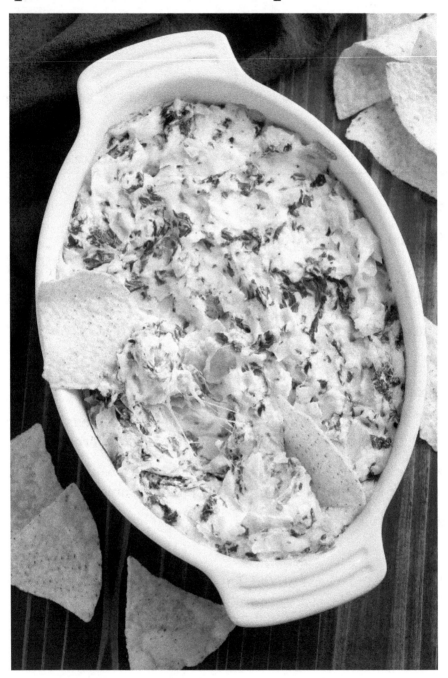

Preparation Time: 10 minutes Cooking Time: 25 minutes Servings: 10

Ingredients:

28 ounces artichokes

1 small white onion, peeled, diced

1 1/2 cups cashews, soaked, drained

4 cups spinach

4 cloves of garlic, peeled

1 1 1/2 teaspoons salt

1/4 cup nutritional yeast

1 tablespoon olive oil

2 tablespoons lemon juice

1 1/2 cups coconut milk, unsweetened

Directions:

1.      Cook onion and garlic in hot oil for 3 minutes until saute and then set aside until required.

2.      Place cashews in a food processor; add 1 teaspoon salt, yeast, milk, and lemon juice and pulse until smooth.

3.      Add spinach, onion mixture, and artichokes and pulse until the chunky mixture comes together.

4.      Tip the dip in a heatproof dish and bake for 20 minutes at 425 degrees f until the top is browned and dip bubbles.

5.      Serve straight away with vegetable sticks.

Nutrition: Calories:124 Cal, Fat: 9 g, Carbs: 8 g, Protein: 5 g, Fiber: 1 g

# Chocolate-Covered Almonds

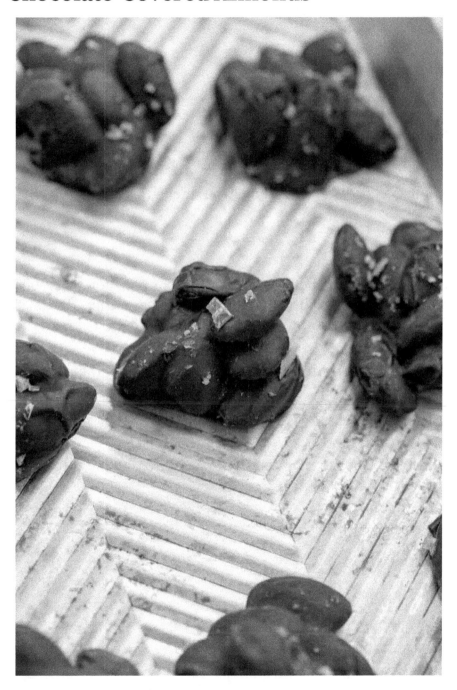

Preparation Time: 1 hour and 45 minutes Cooking Time: 30 seconds

Servings: 4


Ingredients:

8 ounces almonds

1/2 teaspoon sea salt

6 ounces chocolate disks, semisweet, melted


Directions:

1.     Microwave chocolate in a heatproof bowl for 30 seconds until it melts, then dip almonds in it, four at a time, and place them on a baking sheet.

2.     Let almonds stand for 1 hour until hardened, then sprinkle with salt, and cool them in the refrigerator for 30 minutes.

3.     Serve straight away.


Nutrition: Calories:286 Cal, Fat: 22 g, Carbs: 17 g, Protein: 7 g, Fiber: 5 g

# Beans and Spinach Tacos

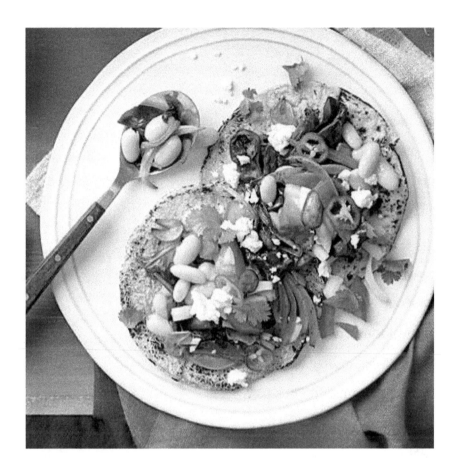

Preparation Time: 10 minutes Cooking Time: 15 minutes

Servings: 4

Ingredients:

12 ounces spinach

4 tablespoons cooked kidney beans

½ of medium red onion, peeled, chopped

½ teaspoon minced garlic

1 medium tomato, chopped

3 tablespoons chopped parsley

½ of avocado, sliced

½ teaspoon ground black pepper

1 teaspoon salt

2 tablespoons olive oil

4 slices of vegan brie cheese

4 tortillas, about 6-inches

Directions:

1.      Take a skillet pan, place it over medium heat, add oil and when hot, add onion and cook for 10 minutes until softened.

2.      Then stir in spinach, cook for 4 minutes until its leaf's wilts, then drain it and distribute evenly between tortillas.

3.     Top evenly with remaining ingredients, season with black pepper and salt, drizzle with lemon juice and then serve.


Nutrition: Calories: 8 Cal, Fat: 6 g, Carbs: 34 g, Protein: 9.9 g, Fiber: 10 g

# Loaded Baked Potatoes

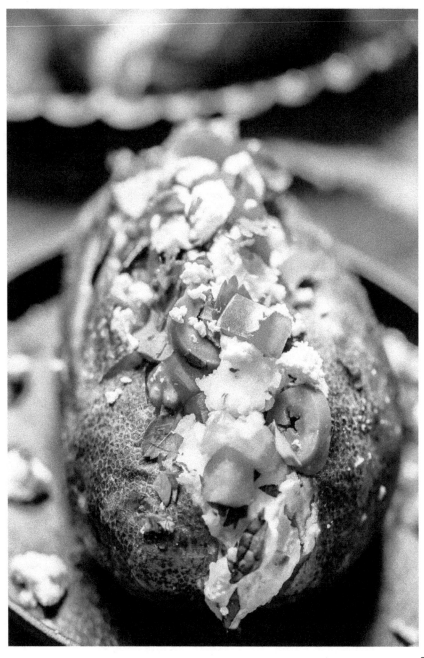

Preparation Time: 10 minutes Cooking Time: 32 minutes Servings: 2

Ingredients:

1/2 cup cooked chickpeas

2 medium potatoes, scrubbed

1 cup broccoli florets, steamed

1/4 cup vegan bacon bits

2 tablespoons all-purpose seasoning

¼ cup vegan cheese sauce

1/2 cup vegan sour cream

Directions:

1.      Pierce hole in the potatoes, microwave them for 12 minutes over high heat setting until soft to touch, and then bake them for 20 minutes at 450 degrees f until very tender.

2.      Open the potatoes, mash the flesh with a fork, then top evenly with remaining ingredients and serve.

Nutrition: Calories: 422 Cal, Fat: 16 g, Carbs: 59 g, Protein: 9 g, Fiber: 6 g

# Coconut Rice

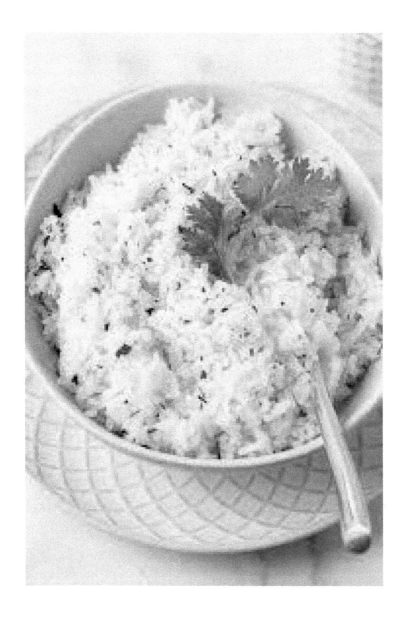

Preparation Time: 5 minutes Cooking Time: 20 minutes Servings: 4

Ingredients:

1 1/2 cups white rice

1 teaspoon coconut sugar

1/8 teaspoon salt

14 ounces coconut milk, unsweetened

1 1/4 cups water

Directions:

1.     Take a saucepan, place it over medium heat, add all the ingredients in it, stir well and bring the mixture to a boil.

2.     Switch heat to medium-low level, simmer the rice for 20 minutes until tender, and then serve straight away.

Nutrition: Calories:453 Cal, Fat: 21 g, Carbs: 61.4 g, Protein: 6.8 g, Fiber: 2 g

# Zucchini and Amaranth Patties

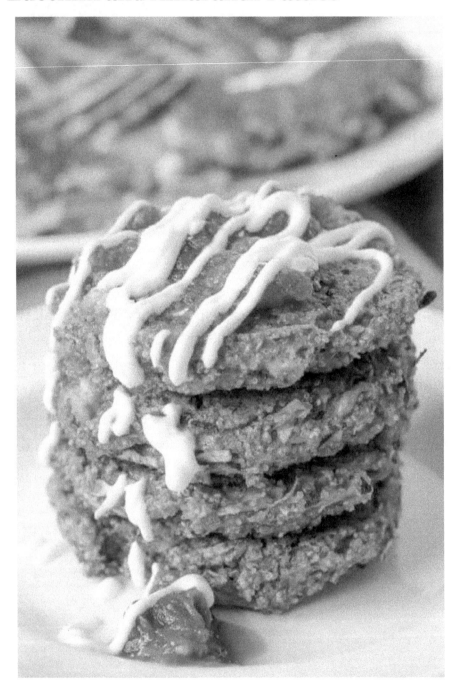

Preparation Time: 10 minutes Cooking Time: 30 minutes Servings: 14

Ingredients:

1 1/2 cups shredded zucchini

½ of a medium onion, shredded

1 1/2 cups cooked white beans

1/2 cup amaranth seeds

1 teaspoon red chili powder

1/2 teaspoon cumin

1/2 cup cornmeal

1/4 cup flax meal

1 tablespoon salsa

1 1/2 cups vegetable broth

Directions:

1.      Stir together stock and amaranth on a pot, bring it to a boil over medium-high heat, then switch heat to medium-low level and simmer until all the liquid is absorbed.

2.      Mash the white beans in a bowl, add remaining ingredients including cooked amaranth and stir until well mixed.

3.      Shape the mixture into patties, then place them on a baking sheet lined with parchment sheet and bake for 30 minutes until browned and crispy, turning halfway.

4.      Serve straight away.

Nutrition: Calories:152 Cal, Fat: 3 g, Carbs: 29 g, Protein: 7 g, Fiber: 6 g

# Rice Pizza

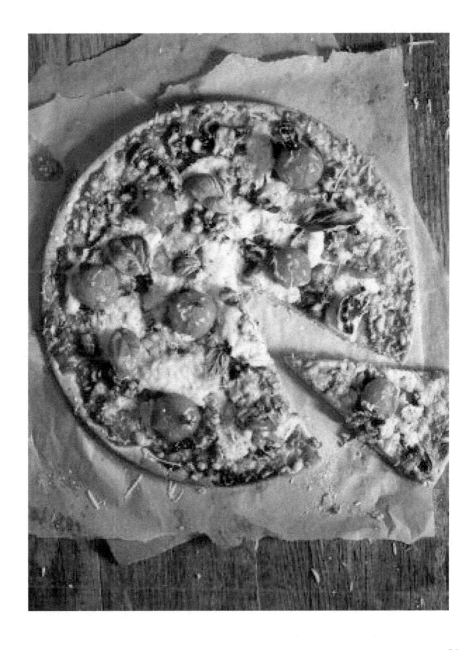

Preparation Time: 10 minutes Cooking Time: 35 minutes
Servings: 6

Ingredients:

For the crust:

1 1/2 cup short-grain rice, cooked

1/2 teaspoon garlic powder

1 teaspoon coconut sugar

1 tablespoon red chili flakes

For the sauce:

1/4 teaspoon onion powder

1        tablespoon nutritional yeast

1/4 teaspoon garlic powder

1/4 teaspoon ginger powder

1 tablespoon red chili flakes

1 teaspoon soy sauce

1/2 cup tomato purée

For the toppings:

2        1/2 cups oyster mushrooms

1 chili pepper, deseeded, sliced

2 scallions, sliced

1 teaspoon coconut sugar

1 teaspoon soy sauce

Baby corn as needed


Directions:

1.      Prepare the crust and for this, place all of its ingredients in a bowl and stir until well combined.

2.      Then take a pizza pan, line it with parchment sheet, place rice mixture in it, spread it evenly, and then bake for 20 minutes at 350 degrees f.

3.      Then spread tomato sauce over the crust, top evenly with remaining ingredients for the topping and continue baking for 15 minutes.

4.      When done, slice the pizza into wedges and serve.


Nutrition: Calories: 1 Cal, Fat: 5 g, Carbs: 30 g, Protein: 3 g, Fiber: 1 g

# Quinoa and Black Bean Burgers

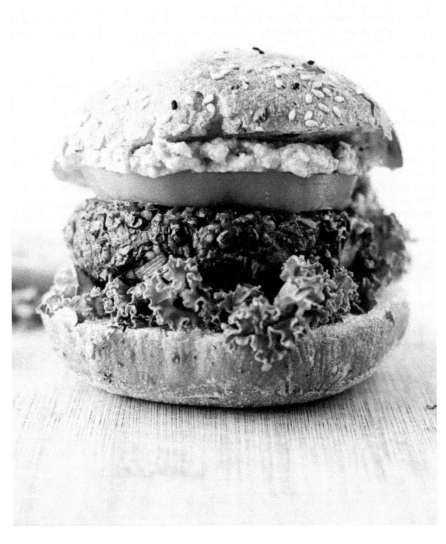

Preparation Time: 10 minutes Cooking Time: 6 minutes Servings: 5

Ingredients:

1/4 cup quinoa, cooked

15 ounces cooked black beans

2 tablespoons minced white onion

1/4 cup minced bell pepper

½ teaspoon minced garlic

1/2 teaspoon salt

1 1/2 teaspoons ground cumin

1/2 cup breadcrumbs

1 teaspoon hot pepper sauce

3 tablespoons olive oil

1 flax egg

Directions:

1.      Place all the ingredients in a bowl, except for oil, stir until well combined, and then shape the mixture into five patties.

2.      Heat oil in a frying pan over medium heat, add patties and cook for 3 minutes per side until browned.

3.      Serve straight away.

Nutrition: Calories: 245 Cal, Fat: 10.6 g, Carbs: 29 g, Protein: 9.3 g, Fiber: 7.2

# Jalapeno and Cilantro Hummus

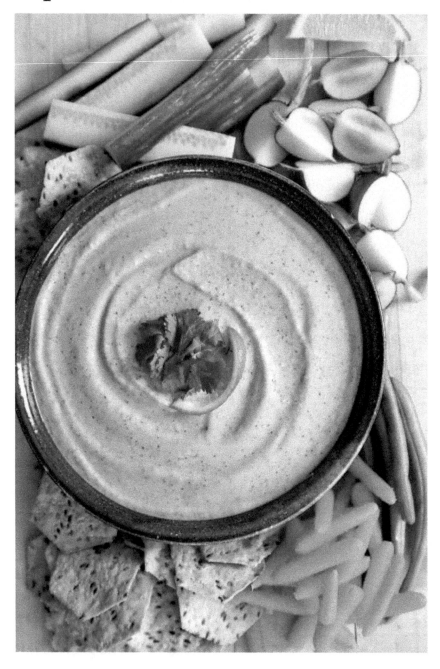

Preparation Time: 5 minutes Cooking Time: 0 minute Servings: 4

Ingredients:

½ cup cilantro

1 1/2 cups chickpeas, cooked

1/2 of jalapeno pepper, sliced

½ teaspoon salt

½ teaspoon minced garlic

1 tablespoon lime juice

1/4 cup tahini

¼ water

Directions:

1.      Place all the ingredients in a bowl and pulse for 2 minutes until smooth.

2.      Tip the hummus in a bowl, drizzle with oil sprinkle with cilantro, and then serve.

Nutrition: Calories: 137 Cal, Fat: 2.3 g, Carbs: 23.3 g, Protein: 7.3 g, Fiber: 6.6 g

# Carrot Cake Bites

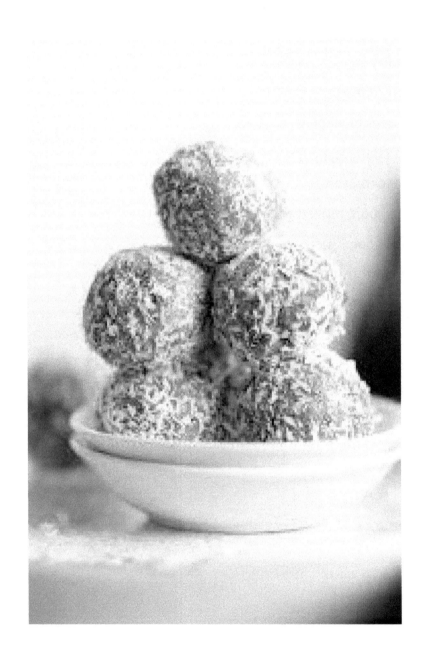

Preparation Time: 15 minutes Cooking Time: 0 minute Servings: 15

Ingredients:

2 cups oats, old-fashioned

½ cup grated carrot

2 cups coconut flakes, unsweetened

1/2 teaspoon salt

1     teaspoon cinnamon

1/2 cup maple syrup

1/2 teaspoon vanilla extract, unsweetened

1/2 cup almond butter

2     tablespoons white chocolate chips

Directions:

1.     Place oats in a food processor, add coconut and pulse until ground.

2.     Then add remaining ingredients except for chocolate chips and pulse for 3 minutes until a sticky dough comes together.

3.     Add chocolate chips, pulse for 1 minute until just mixed, and then shape the mixture into fifteen small balls.

4.     Refrigerate the balls for 30 minutes and then serve.

Nutrition: Calories: 87 Cal, Fat: 5 g, Carbs: 9.2 g, Protein: 1.8 g, Fiber: 1.6 g

# Cinnamon Bun Balls

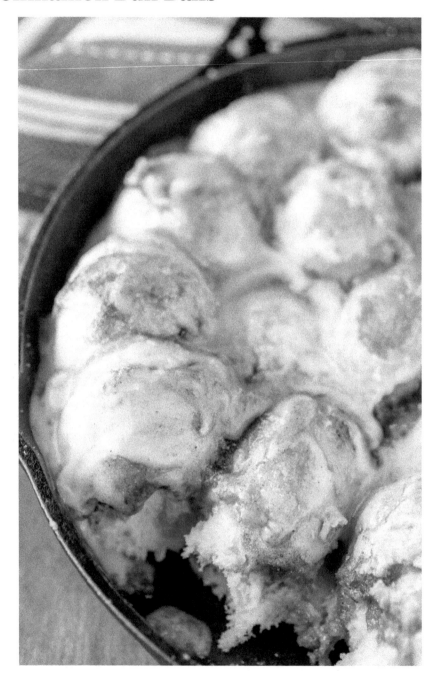

Preparation Time: 15 minutes Cooking Time: 0 minute Servings: 10

Ingredients:

5 medjool dates, pitted

1/2 cup whole walnuts

1        tablespoon chopped walnuts

3 tablespoons ground cinnamon

1 teaspoon ground cardamom

Directions:

1.       Place all the ingredients in a food processor, except for 1 tablespoon walnuts, and then process until smooth.

2.       Shape the mixture into ten balls, then roll them into chopped walnuts and serve.

Nutrition: Calories:62 Cal, Fat: 4.5 g, Carbs: 5.8 g, Protein: 1.2 g, Fiber: 2 g

# Kale Hummus

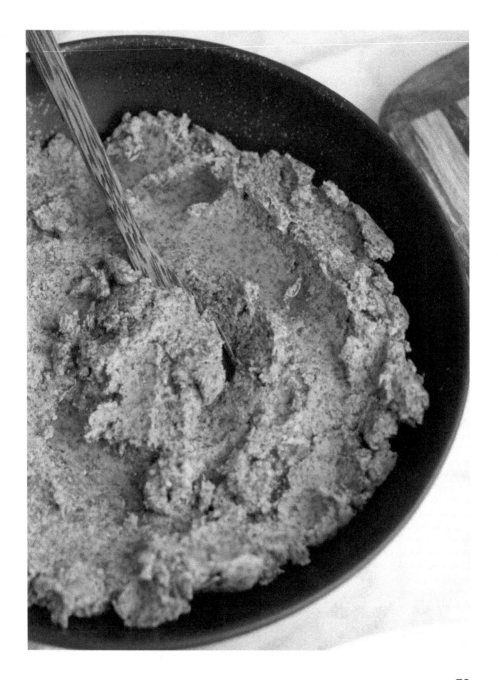

Preparation Time: 5 minutes Cooking Time: 0 minute Servings: 4

Ingredients:

2      cups cooked chickpeas

5 cloves of garlic, peeled

4 cups kale, torn into pieces

1 teaspoon of sea salt

1/3 cup lemon juice

1/4 cup olive oil

1/4 cup tahini

Directions:

1.      Place all the ingredients in a bowl and pulse for 2 minutes until smooth.

2.      Tip the hummus in a bowl, drizzle with oil, and then serve.

Nutrition: Calories: 173 Cal, Fat: 10 g, Carbs: 14 g, Protein: 6 g, Fiber: 5 g

# Zesty Orange-Cranberry Energy Bites

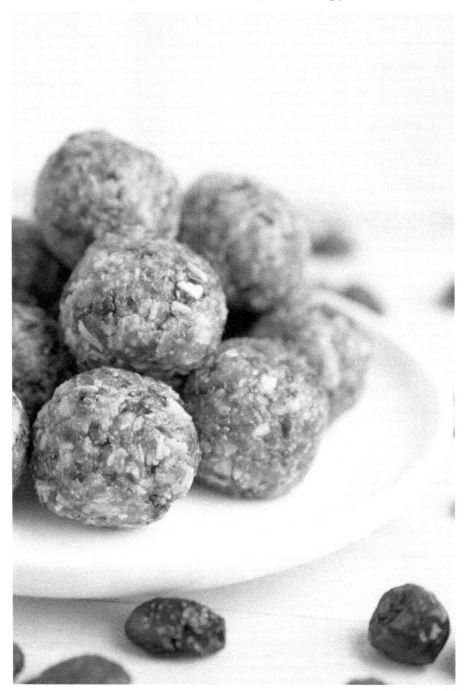

Preparation Time: 10 minutes Chill Time: 15 minutes Serves: 12 bites

Ingredients:

2 tablespoons almond butter, or cashew or sunflower seed butter
2 tablespoons maple syrup, or brown rice syrup

¾ cup cooked quinoa

¼ cup sesame seeds, toasted

1 tablespoon chia seeds

½ teaspoon almond extract, or vanilla extract

Zest of 1 orange

1 tablespoon dried cranberries

¼ cup ground almonds

Directions:

1.      In a medium bowl, mix together the nut or seed butter and syrup until smooth and creamy. Stir in the rest of the ingredients, and mix to make sure the consistency is holding together in a ball. Form the mix into 12 balls.

2.      Place them on a baking sheet lined with parchment or waxed paper and put in the fridge to set for about 15 minutes.

3.      If your balls aren't holding together, it's likely because of the moisture content of your cooked quinoa.

4.      Add more nut or seed butter mixed with syrup until it all sticks together.

Nutrition (1 bite): Calories: 109; total fat: 7g, Carbs: 11g, Fiber: 3g, Protein: 3g

# Chocolate Melt Chaffles

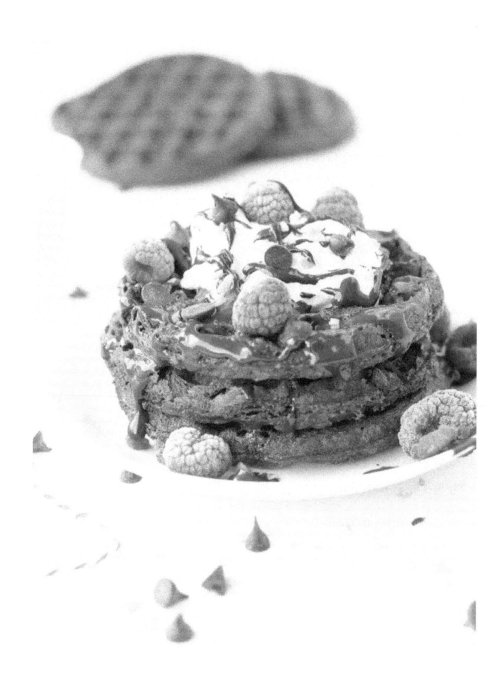

Preparation Time: 15 minutes Cooking Time: 36 minutes Servings: 4

Ingredients:

For the chaffles:

2 eggs, beaten

¼ cup finely grated Gruyere cheese

2 tbsp heavy cream

1 tbsp coconut flour

2 tbsp cream cheese, softened

3 tbsp unsweetened cocoa powder

2 tsp vanilla extract

A pinch of salt

For the chocolate sauce:

1/3 cup + 1 tbsp heavy cream

1 ½ oz unsweetened baking chocolate, chopped

1 ½ tsp sugar-free maple syrup

1 ½ tsp vanilla extract

Directions:

For the chaffles:

1. Preheat the cast iron pan.

2. In a medium bowl, mix all the ingredients for the chaffles.

3.      Open the iron and add a quarter of the mixture. Close and cook until crispy, 7 minutes.

4.      Transfer the chaffle to a plate and make 3 more with the remaining batter. For the chocolate sauce:

5.      Pour the heavy cream into saucepan and simmer over low heat, 3 minutes.

6.      Turn the heat off and add the chocolate. Allow melting for a few minutes and stir until fully melted, 5 minutes.

7.      Mix in the maple syrup and vanilla extract.

8.      Assemble the chaffles in layers with the chocolate sauce sandwiched between each layer.

9.      Slice and serve immediately.


Nutrition: Calories 172, Fats 13.57g, Carbs 6.65g, Net Carbs 3.65g, Protein 5.76g

# Chaffles With Keto Ice Cream

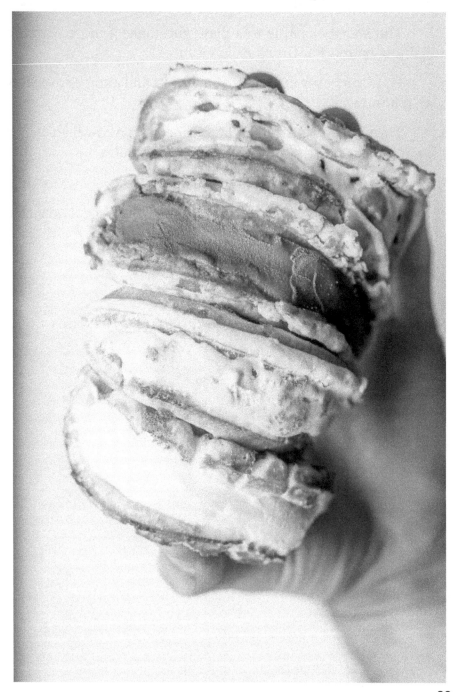

Preparation Time: 10 minutes Cooking Time: 14 minutes Servings: 2

Ingredients:

1       egg, beaten

½ cup finely grated mozzarella cheese

¼ cup almond flour

2       tbsp swerve confectioner's sugar

1/8 tsp xanthan gum

Low-carb ice cream (flavor of your choice) for serving

Directions:

1.      Preheat the cast iron pan.

2.      In a medium bowl, mix all the ingredients except the ice cream.

3.      Open the iron and add half of the mixture. Close and cook until crispy, 7 minutes.

4.      Transfer the chaffle to a plate and make second one with the remaining batter.

5.      On each chaffle, add a scoop of low carb ice cream, fold into half-moons and enjoy.

Nutrition: Calories 89, Fats 6.48g, Carbs 1.67g, Net Carbs 1.37g, Protein 5.91g

# Strawberry Shortcake Chaffle Bowls

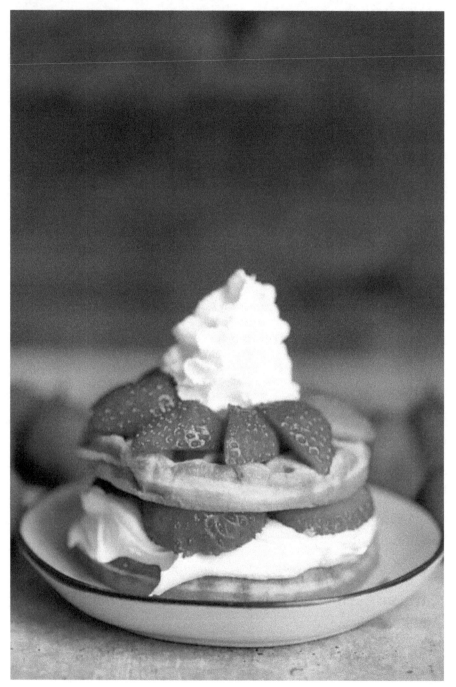

Preparation Time: 10 minutes Cooking Time: 28 minutes Servings: 4

Ingredients:

1        egg, beaten

½ cup finely grated mozzarella cheese

1 tbsp almond flour

¼ tsp baking powder

2        drops cake batter extract

1 cup cream cheese, softened

1 cup fresh strawberries, sliced

1 tbsp sugar-free maple syrup

Directions:

1.      Preheat the cast iron pan.

2.      Meanwhile, in a medium bowl, whisk all the ingredients except the cream cheese and strawberries.

3.      Open the iron, pour in half of the mixture, cover, and cook until crispy, 6 to 7 minutes.

4.      Remove the chaffle bowl onto a plate and set aside.

5.      Make a second chaffle bowl with the remaining batter.

6.      To serve, divide the cream cheese into the chaffle bowls and top with the strawberries.

7.      Drizzle the filling with the maple syrup and serve.

Nutrition: Calories 235, Fats 20.62g, Carbs 5.9g, Net Carbs 5g, Protein 7.51g

# Chaffles With Raspberry Syrup

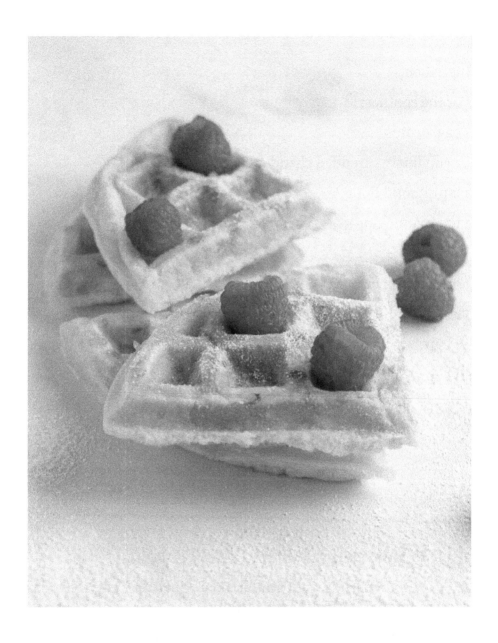

Preparation Time: 10 minutes Cooking Time: 38 minutes

Servings: 4

Ingredients:

For the chaffles:

1 egg, beaten

½ cup finely shredded cheddar cheese

1 tsp almond flour

1 tsp sour cream

For the raspberry syrup:

1 cup fresh raspberries

¼ cup swerve sugar

¼ cup water

1 tsp vanilla extract

Directions:

For the chaffles:

1.      Preheat the cast iron pan.

2.      Meanwhile, in a medium bowl, mix the egg, cheddar cheese, almond flour, and sour cream.

3.      Open the iron, pour in half of the mixture, cover, and cook until crispy, 7 minutes.

4.    Remove the chaffle onto a plate and make another with the remaining batter. For the raspberry syrup:

5.    Meanwhile, add the raspberries, swerve sugar, water, and vanilla extract to a medium pot. Set over low heat and cook until the raspberries soften and sugar becomes syrupy. Occasionally stir while mashing the raspberries as you go. Turn the heat off when your desired consistency is achieved and set aside to cool.

6.    Drizzle some syrup on the chaffles and enjoy when ready.

Nutrition: Calories 105, Fats 7.11g, Carbs 4.31g, Net Carbs 2.21g, Protein 5.83g

# Chaffle Cannoli

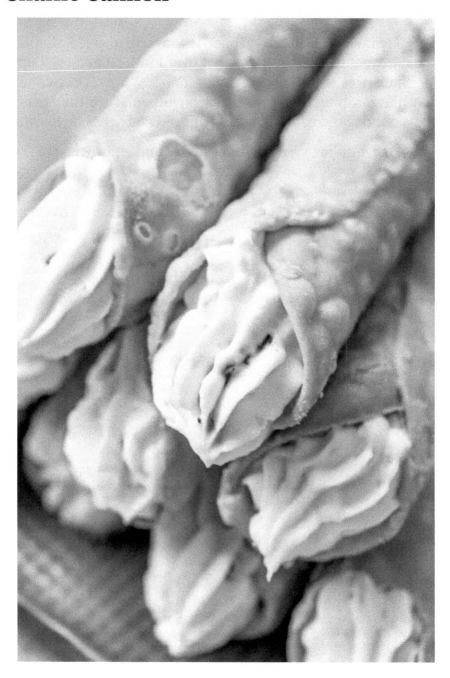

Preparation Time: 15 minutes Cooking Time: 28 minutes Servings: 4

Ingredients:

For the chaffles:

1 large egg

1 egg yolk

3 tbsp butter, melted

1 tbso swerve confectioner's

1      cup finely grated Parmesan cheese

2 tbsp finely grated mozzarella cheese

For the cannoli filling:

½ cup ricotta cheese

2      tbsp swerve confectioner's sugar 1 tsp vanilla extract

2 tbsp unsweetened chocolate chips for garnishing

Directions:

1.      Preheat the cast iron pan.

2.      Meanwhile, in a medium bowl, mix all the ingredients for the chaffles.

3.      Open the iron, pour in a quarter of the mixture, cover, and cook until crispy, 7 minutes.

4.      Remove the chaffle onto a plate and make 3 more with the remaining batter.

5.      Meanwhile, for the cannoli filling:

6.      Beat the ricotta cheese and swerve confectioner's sugar until smooth. Mix in the vanilla.

7.      On each chaffle, spread some of the filling and wrap over.

8.      Garnish the creamy ends with some chocolate chips.

9.      Serve immediately.


Nutrition: Calories 308, Fats 25.05g, Carbs 5.17g, Net Carbs 5.17g, Protein 15.18g

# Orange Polenta Cake

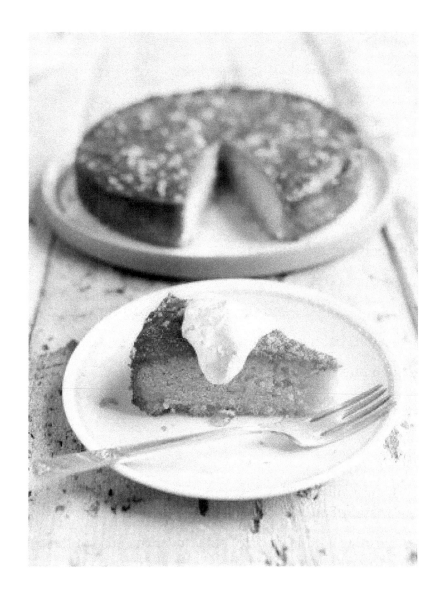

Preparation Time: 30 Minutes Servings: 6

Ingredients:

1¼ cups all-purpose flour

1 cup unsweetened almond milk

2/3 cup plus

1 tablespoon natural sugar

⅓ cup fine-ground cornmeal

⅓ cup plus 2 tablespoons marmalade

¼ cup finely ground almonds

¼ cup vegan butter, softened

1 navel orange, peeled and sliced into ⅛-inch-thick rounds

1½ teaspoons baking powder

1 teaspoon pure vanilla extract

¾ teaspoon salt

Directions:

1.      Lightly oil a baking tray that will fit in the steamer basket of your Instant Pot.

2.      Sprinkle a tablespoon of sugar over the base of the baking tray and top with the orange slices.

3.      In a bowl combine the flour, cornmeal, baking powder, almonds, and salt.

4. In another bowl combine the remaining sugar, the butter, 1/3 cup of marmalade, and vanilla and mix well. Slowly stir in the almond milk.

5. Combine the wet and dry mixes into a smooth batter.

6. Pour the batter into your baking tray and put the tray in your steamer basket.

7. Pour the minimum amount of water into the base of your Instant Pot and lower the steamer basket.

8. Seal and cook on Steam for 12 minutes.

9. Release the pressure quickly and set to one side to cool a little.

10. Warm the remaining 2 tablespoons of marmalade and brush over the cake.

# Peanut Butter & Chocolate Cheesecake.

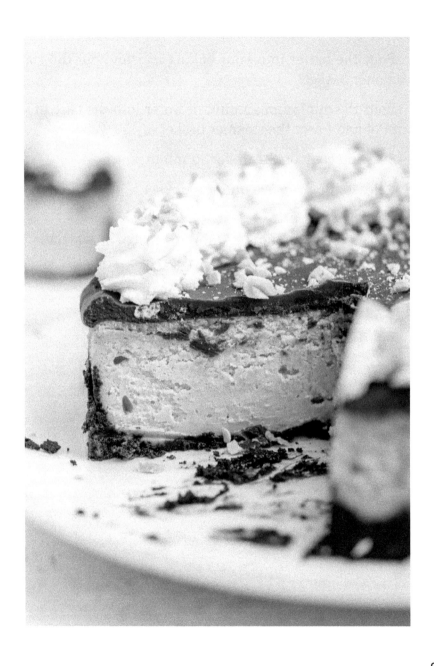

Preparation Time: 30 Minutes Servings: 8

Ingredients:

16 ounces vegan cream cheese

8 ounces silken tofu, drained

1½ cups crushed vegan chocolate cookies

¾ cup natural sugar

½ cup creamy peanut butter, at room temperature

¼ cup unsweetened cocoa powder

3 tablespoons vegan butter, melted

2 tablespoons hazelnut milk

Directions:

1.     Lightly oil a baking tray that will fit in the steamer basket of your Instant Pot.

2.     Combine the chocolate crumbs and the butter.

3.     Press the chocolate base into your tray.

4.     Blend the cream cheese and tofu until smooth.

5.     Add the peanut butter, cocoa, hazelnut milk, and sugar to the cheese mix and fold in well.

6.     Pour the cheese onto your base and put the tray in your steamer basket.

7.     Pour the minimum amount of water into the base of your Instant Pot and lower the steamer basket.

8.     Seal and cook on Steam for 15 minutes.

9.　　Release the pressure quickly and set to one side to cool a little.

# Blueberry Brownies

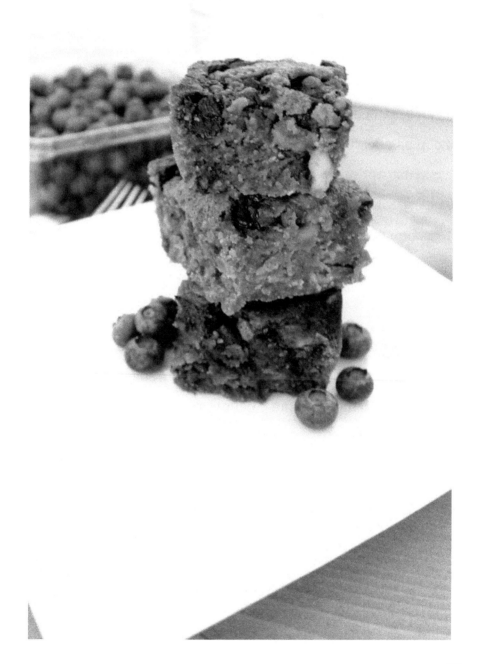

Preparation Time: 20 Minutes Servings: 8

Ingredients:

1      cup cooked black beans

¾ cup unbleached all-purpose flour

½ cup unsweetened cocoa powder

½ cup blueberry jam

½ cup natural sugar

1½ teaspoons baking powder

1 teaspoon pure vanilla extract

Directions:

1.     Lightly oil a baking tray that will fit in the steamer basket of your Instant Pot.

2.     Blend together the beans, cocoa, jam, sugar, and vanilla.

3.     Fold in the flour and baking powder until the batter is smooth.

4.     Pour the batter into your tray and put the tray in your steamer basket.

5.     Pour the minimum amount of water into the base of your Instant Pot and lower the steamer basket.

6.     Seal and cook on Steam for 12 minutes.

7.     Release the pressure quickly and set to one side to cool a little before slicing.

# Pumpkin Spice Oat Bars

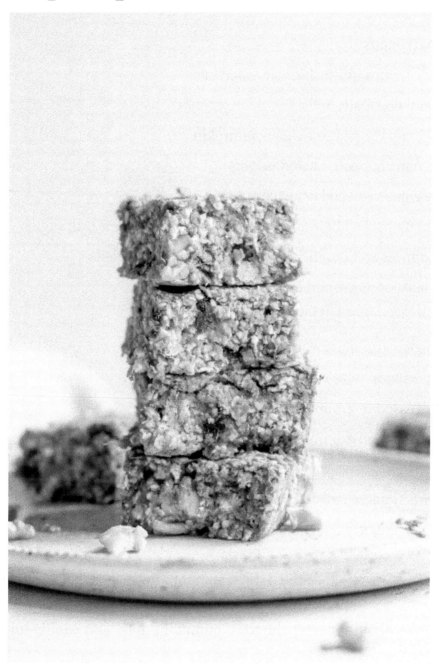

Preparation Time: 25 Minutes Servings: 10

Ingredients:

2      cups old-fashioned rolled oats

1 cup non-dairy milk

2/3 cup canned solid-pack pumpkin

½ cup chopped toasted pecans

½ cup sweetened dried cranberries

½ cup packed light brown sugar or granulated natural sugar

6 ounces soft or silken tofu, drained and crumbled

2 teaspoons ground cinnamon

1½ teaspoons baking powder

1 teaspoon salt

1 teaspoon pure vanilla extract

¼ teaspoon ground nutmeg

¼ teaspoon ground allspice

Directions:

1.     Lightly oil a baking tray that will fit in the steamer basket of your Instant Pot.

2.     Stir together the oats, cinnamon, nutmeg, allspice, sugar, baking powder, and salt.

3.     Blend together the tofu, pumpkin, milk, and vanilla until smooth and even.

4.      Stir the wet and dry ingredients together before folding in the pecans and cranberries.

5.      Pour the batter into your tray and put the tray in your steamer basket.

6.      Pour the minimum amount of water into the base of your Instant Pot and lower the steamer basket.

7.      Seal and cook on Steam for 12 minutes.

8.      Release the pressure quickly and set to one side to cool a little before slicing.

# Tutti Frutti Cobbler

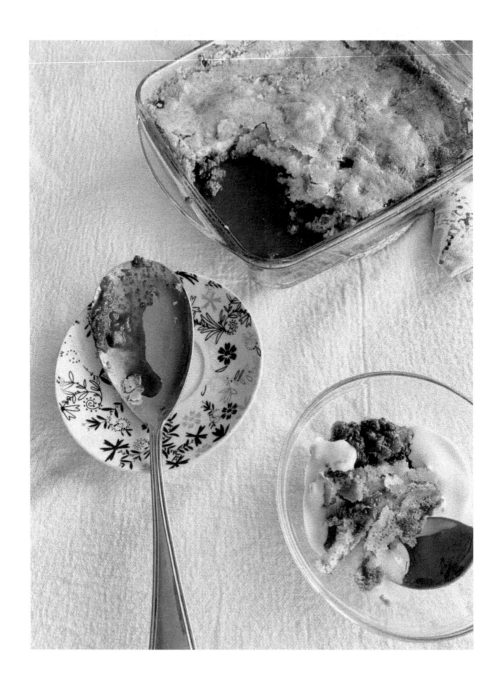

Preparation Time: 30 Minutes Servings: 6

Ingredients:

1¼ cups unbleached all-purpose flour

1      cup fresh blueberries, rinsed and picked over

1 cup fresh blackberries, rinsed and picked over

¾ cup natural sugar

½ cup unsweetened almond milk

2      large ripe peaches, peeled, pitted, and sliced

2 ripe apricots, peeled, pitted, and sliced

1½ tablespoons tapioca starch or cornstarch

1 tablespoon vegetable oil

1 teaspoon baking powder

½ teaspoon pure vanilla extract

¼ teaspoon salt

¼ teaspoon ground cinnamon

Directions:

1.     Lightly oil a baking tray that will fit in the steamer basket of your Instant Pot.

2.     Toss the fruit in the tapioca and ½ a cup of sugar and put in the tray.

3.     Put the tray in your steamer basket.

4.    Pour the minimum amount of water into the base of your Instant Pot and lower the steamer basket.

5.    Seal and cook on Steam for 12 minutes.

6.    In a bowl stir together the flour, remaining sugar, cinnamon, baking powder, and salt.

7.    Slowly combine with the almond milk, vanilla, and oil until soft dough is formed.

8.    Release the Instant Pot's pressure quickly, give the fruit a stir, and cover with the dough.

9.    Seal and Steam for another 5 minutes.

10.    Release the pressure quickly and set to one side to cool a little.

# Pear Mincemeat

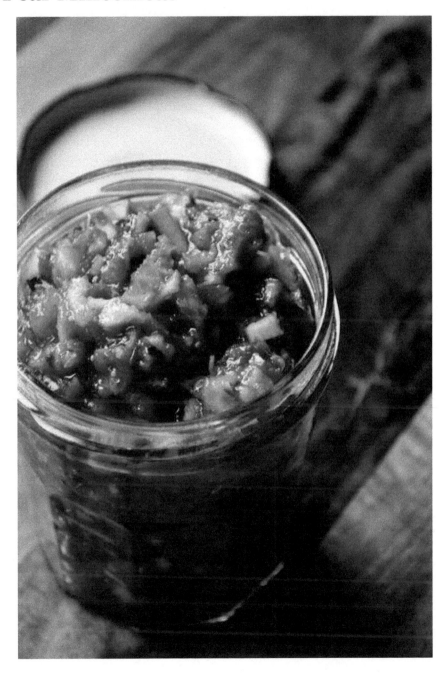

Preparation Time: 35 Minutes Servings: 6

Ingredients:

4 firm ripe Bosc pears, peeled, cored, and chopped

1 large orange

1½ cups apple juice

1¼ cups granola of your choice

1 cup raisins (dark, golden, or a combination

1 cup chopped dried apples, pears, or apricots, or a combination

½ cup packed dark brown sugar or granulated natural sugar

¼ cup brandy or 1 teaspoon brandy extract

2 tablespoons pure maple syrup or agave nectar

2 tablespoons cider vinegar

½ teaspoon ground cinnamon

½ teaspoon ground allspice

½ teaspoon ground nutmeg

¼ teaspoon ground cloves

Pinch of salt

Directions:

1. Zest the orange, then peel it, deseed it, and quarter it.

2. Blend the orange flesh and zest and put in your Instant Pot.

3.    Add the pears, dried fruits, juice, sugar, brandy spices, vinegar, and salt.

4.    Seal and cook on Stew for 12 minutes.

5.    Release the pressure naturally, take out some of the juice, then reseal and cook another 12 minutes.

6.    In a bowl mix the granola and syrup.

7.    Release the pressure of the Instant Pot naturally and sprinkle the crumble on top.

8.    Seal the Instant Pot and cook on Stew for another 5 minutes.

9.    Release the pressure naturally and serve.

# Apple & Walnut Cake

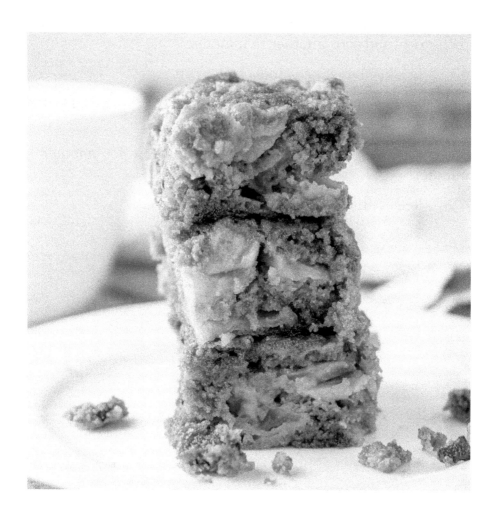

Preparation Time: 20 Minutes Servings: 6

Ingredients:

1¾ cups unbleached all-purpose flour

1 cup unsweetened applesauce

⅔ cup packed light brown sugar

½ cup chopped walnuts

¼ cup vegetable oil

1        tablespoon freshly squeezed lemon juice

1 teaspoon pure vanilla extract

1½ teaspoons ground cinnamon

1 teaspoon baking powder

½ teaspoon baking soda

½ teaspoon salt

¼ teaspoon ground allspice

¼ teaspoon ground nutmeg

⅛ teaspoon ground cloves


Directions:

1.      Lightly oil a baking tray that will fit in the steamer basket of your Instant Pot.

2.      In a bowl, combine the flour, baking powder, baking soda, sugar, cinnamon, allspice, nutmeg, cloves, and salt.

3.     In another bowl combine the applesauce, oil, vanilla, and lemon juice.

4.     Stir the wet mixture into the dry mixture slowly until they form a smooth mix.

5.     Fold in the walnuts.

6.     Pour the batter into your baking tray and put the tray in your steamer basket.

7.     Pour the minimum amount of water into the base of your Instant Pot and lower the steamer basket.

8.     Seal and cook on Steam for 12 minutes.

9.     Release the pressure quickly and set to one side to cool a little.

Lightning Source UK Ltd.
Milton Keynes UK
UKHW020952070521
383312UK00013B/986